Simplified Solution Approach
To **GLAUCOMA**

Illuminating Perspectives: A Comprehensive
Approach to Elevate Your Visual Wellbeing
and Embrace a World of Limitless Clarity

Dr QUENTIN GLYN

Table Of Contents

CHAPTER ONE
Glaucoma

A class of eye conditions known as glaucoma is defined by damage to the optic nerve and is often linked to elevated intraocular pressure (IOP). It is one of the main causes of permanent blindness around the globe. This article emphasizes the need for early identification for successful therapy of glaucoma and offers a simple way to understand the condition.

Definition:

A group of eye disorders known as glaucoma causes damage to the optic nerve, which in turn causes vision loss. For visual information to be sent from the eye to the brain, the optic nerve is essential. Primary open-angle glaucoma (POAG), the most prevalent kind of glaucoma, is characterized by a progressive rise in intraocular pressure. Angle-closure glaucoma and normal-tension glaucoma are two further types.

Frequency And Effects:

Millions of people worldwide suffer from the common eye condition glaucoma. Over 76 million individuals worldwide are estimated to have glaucoma by the World Health Organization (WHO), and this figure is predicted to increase dramatically in the years to come. Given that glaucoma may result in irreversible visual loss and a worse quality of life, it has a significant effect on both people and society.

The Value Of Early Identification:

It is essential to identify glaucoma early for a number of reasons:

1. Quiet Advancement:

When glaucoma first develops, it often advances quietly and shows no symptoms at all. It is possible that permanent harm has already happened by the time symptoms show up. Frequent eye examinations, which include optic nerve assessment and tonometry (measurement of intraocular pressure), may identify glaucoma early on.

2. Preventing Permanent Damage:

The harm glaucoma causes to the visual nerve cannot be reversed. On the other hand, the disease's course may be slowed down or stopped by early discovery and proper intervention, such as medication or surgery, avoiding further loss of vision.

3. Maintenance of Life Quality:

The everyday activities and freedom of a person may be greatly impacted by vision loss resulting from glaucoma. Early identification enables prompt care, keeping functional eyesight and protecting the person's quality of life.

4. Expense-effectiveness:

Treating glaucoma at late stages of the illness is more expensive than early identification and care. Routine eye exams are an easy and affordable way to detect glaucoma early on, which lowers the financial burden of late-stage treatments.

5. Impact on Public Health:

Proactive glaucoma screening reduces the total societal burden of blindness and is consistent with public health efforts. Increased early detection and better results may be attained by screening programs, education, and awareness initiatives.

In conclusion, tackling this serious public health concern requires an awareness of the fundamentals of glaucoma and the need for early identification. Frequent eye exams are essential for detecting glaucoma early on, which allows for prompt intervention and the preservation of vision and quality of life, particularly for those who are more vulnerable.

Through raising awareness and taking preventative action, we may try to lessen the effects of glaucoma on people and the community.

CHAPTER TWO

Comprehending Glaucoma

A class of eye diseases known as glaucoma harms the optic nerve, which is essential for clear vision. Increased intraocular pressure (IOP) is often the source of the injury, although it may also happen with normal or even lower-than-normal IOP. Glaucoma may cause blindness and irreversible visual loss if treatment is not received.

The Eye's Anatomy:

The eye is a multifaceted organ made up of several important parts. The transparent front surface of the eye that lets light in is called the cornea. The colorful portion of the eye that controls how much light enters is called the iris.

The retina, a tissue in the back of the eye that is sensitive to light, receives light focus from the lens. The optic nerve connects the retina to the brain, carrying visual information. Gaining an understanding of these elements is crucial to understanding how glaucoma impacts vision.

Intraocular Pressure Mechanisms:

The fluid pressure within the eye is known as intraocular pressure or IOP. Aqueous humor, a transparent fluid produced by the eye, has to drain appropriately to keep the intraocular pressure (IOP) at a healthy range. IOP may rise and cause glaucoma if the drainage is blocked or if the eye generates too much fluid. To keep the pressure in the eyes at normal levels, the production and drainage of aqueous humor must be balanced.

Glaucoma Types:

Angle-Opening Glaucoma:

This kind of glaucoma is the most prevalent. The drainage angle where the iris and cornea meet is open in open-angle glaucoma, but it gradually loses efficiency. The optic nerve may be harmed by this slow decrease in outflow, which may raise IOP.

Glaucoma with an angle closure:

Angle-closure glaucoma, in contrast to open-angle glaucoma, is caused by a blockage or covering of the drainage angle, which stops aqueous humor from draining. This may lead to an abrupt rise in IOP, which might produce acute symptoms including excruciating headaches, impaired vision, and eye discomfort. Angle-closure glaucoma is regarded as an urgent medical condition.

Untensioned Glaucoma:

Even when IOP is within the usual range, optic nerve damage happens in normal-tension glaucoma. Although the precise etiology is unknown, potential contributing variables include inadequate blood supply to the optic nerve and an enhanced sensitivity of the optic nerve to normal intraocular pressure levels.

Simplified Method Of Solving:

Frequent ocular examinations:

Promote regular ocular examinations to identify early indicators of glaucoma.

For vision loss to be managed and prevented, early diagnosis is essential.

Consciousness and Instruction:

Raise public knowledge of glaucoma, its contributing causes, and the need for routine eye exams.

Inform them about the several forms of glaucoma and the function of IOP.

Changes in Lifestyle:

Stress leads to a healthy lifestyle that includes frequent exercise and a well-balanced diet.

Some exercises, such as yoga, may assist in controlling intraocular pressure and enhancing general eye health.

Adherence to Medication:

If a diagnosis is made, emphasize how crucial it is to take prescription drugs as directed.

Certain drugs lower intraocular pressure (IOP) by either enhancing drainage or reducing fluid generation.

Surgical Procedures:

If medicine is not enough, surgical procedures could be taken into consideration.

Surgical techniques or laser treatment may enhance fluid outflow.

Frequent Check-ins:

Emphasize the need to schedule regular follow-up visits to track the development of glaucoma and modify therapy as necessary.

Support Groups for Patients:

Create or suggest glaucoma support groups for affected persons.

Shared experiences and emotional support might be helpful in managing the illness.

To summarize, a straightforward strategy for treating glaucoma entails raising awareness, identifying the condition early, changing one's lifestyle, taking medicine as prescribed, and, if required, undergoing surgery. An important element of this plan to prevent or reduce vision loss related to glaucoma is patient education and routine eye exams.

CHAPTER THREE

Symptoms And Risk Factors

A class of eye diseases known as glaucoma may harm the optic nerve; this is usually the result of high intraocular pressure (IOP). It is one of the main causes of permanent blindness around the globe. Let's examine the glaucoma risk factors and symptoms in order to streamline the remedy strategy.

Hazardous Elements

1. Age:

Reason: The risk of glaucoma rises with age, and those over 60 are more likely to get it.

Simplified Approach: To identify and treat glaucoma early, people over 60 must have regular eye exams.

2. Family Background:

Explanation: The risk is increased if glaucoma runs in the family.

Simplified Approach: Having knowledge of your family history aids in proactive screening, allowing for any required early action.

3. Ethnicity

Justification: There is an increased danger for some ethnic groups, including Asians, Hispanics, and African Americans.

Simplified Approach: People who belong to high-risk ethnic groups should schedule regular eye checkups and be more mindful of their eye health.

4. Health Issues:

Justification: Heart disease, high blood pressure, and diabetes may all raise the risk.

Simplified Approach: Maintaining general health lowers the chance of developing glaucoma, highlighting the need to lead a healthy lifestyle.

Signs:

1. Vision Shifts:

Justification: One typical sign is a progressive loss of peripheral vision.

Simplified Approach: Frequent eye examinations or regular self-checks for abnormalities in peripheral vision aid in early identification.

2. Redness and Pain in the Eyes:

Explanation: Acute glaucoma patients may experience intense eye discomfort and redness.

Simplified Approach: If you experience sudden redness and discomfort in your eyes, you should seek medical assistance right away since this might be a sign of an acute glaucoma episode.

3. Loss of Peripheral Vision:

Reason: Gradual loss of peripheral vision, often undetectable until a substantial loss happens.

Simplified Approach: Early detection of peripheral vision loss is facilitated by routine eye examinations, even in the absence of symptoms.

A simple method of treating glaucoma relies heavily on diagnosing symptoms and comprehending risk factors. Frequent ocular examinations are essential, particularly for those who are elderly, have a family history of eye disorders, are members of a certain ethnic group, or have underlying medical diseases. By identifying minor indicators like as changes in vision and being alert for unexpected discomfort or redness, one may effectively treat and diagnose glaucoma early on, lowering the chance of permanent vision loss.

CHAPTER FOUR
Methods Of Diagnosis

A class of eye diseases known as glaucoma may harm the optic nerve, which, if unchecked, can result in blindness and visual loss. Several diagnostic methods are used to diagnose and track glaucoma since early identification is essential for efficient treatment. Below is a detailed summary of the main diagnostic methods:

Full-Service Eye Exam:

Glaucoma diagnosis begins with a thorough eye examination. It entails a comprehensive evaluation of the patient's medical background, family history, and ocular examination.

A standard eye exam includes evaluating visual acuity, inspecting the cornea, lens, and retina, and looking for anomalies in the optic nerve head.

Using eye drops to dilate the pupils enables a closer look at the retinal nerve fiber layer and the optic nerve head.

Measuring Intraocular Pressure:

The risk of developing glaucoma is significantly increased intraocular pressure (IOP). The instrument used to measure IOP is tonometry.

The most popular kind of tonometry is called "Goldmann applanation tonometry," in which a tonometer is used to apply a little amount of pressure to the cornea. This gauges the amount of force needed to flatten a particular corneal region.

Although elevated IOP by itself does not prove glaucoma, it is a significant consideration in the evaluation process.

Visual Field Examination:

Peripheral vision loss is a common side effect of glaucoma that might be missed in its early stages. To find these flaws, visual field testing is essential.

The most used visual field test is perimetry. When the patient notices lights in their peripheral vision, they signal and fix their attention on a central location. This aids in mapping the visual field.

Because automated perimetry is accurate and repeatable, it is often utilized. One example of this is the Humphrey Visual Field Test.

OCT, or optical coherence tomography,

High-resolution cross-sectional pictures of the optic nerve head, retina, and retinal nerve fiber layer may be obtained using OCT, a non-invasive imaging method.

It aids in determining the retinal nerve fiber layer's thickness, which may be a sign of glaucomatous damage.

OCT is helpful for tracking changes over time and is especially helpful for glaucoma early detection.

Gonioscopy:

A specialist test called a gonioscopy is used to measure the eye's drainage angle, which is important to comprehend the mechanism behind raised intraocular pressure (IOP) in certain forms of glaucoma.

After applying a certain gel or solution to the cornea, a goniolens is positioned there. This makes it possible to see the angle that forms between the iris and cornea directly.

It assists in identifying whether the angle is open, narrow, or closed, providing crucial details for the diagnosis and treatment of different kinds of glaucoma.

To sum up, a variety of methods are used to diagnose glaucoma, including clinical assessment, tonometry, visual field tests, imaging modalities like OCT, and specialist procedures like gonioscopy. In order to effectively treat glaucoma and preserve the patient's eyesight and quality of life, early identification and ongoing monitoring are crucial.

CHAPTER FIVE
Options For Current Treatment

A class of eye diseases known as glaucoma may harm the optic nerve, resulting in blindness or visual loss. Since increased intraocular pressure (IOP) is a major risk factor for the advancement of glaucoma, the primary objective of therapy is to lower IOP. This is a comprehensive summary of the glaucoma treatments available today:

Drugs:

Eye Drops:

The most popular first glaucoma therapy is eye drops. They function by either boosting the drainage of the eye's aqueous humor or decreasing its production. Typical varieties of eye drops consist of:

1. Analogs of prostaglandins: These stimulate the release of aqueous humor. Bimatoprost, travoprost, and latanoprost are a few examples.

2. Beta-blockers: They lessen the aqueous humor produced. One often used beta-blocker is Timolol.

3. Alpha agonists: These cause the generation of aqueous humor to decrease while its drainage increases. Praclonidine and brimonidine are two examples.

4. Inhibitors of carbonic anhydrase: They reduce the generation of watery humor.

Examples are brinzolamide and dorzolamide.

Oral Drugs:

Oral drugs may be recommended in certain circumstances in order to regulate intraocular pressure. Oral carbonic anhydrase inhibitors, including acetazolamide, are often utilized.

Laser Treatment:

Trabeculoplasty using Selective Laser (SLT):

Using a laser, SLT improves drainage and lowers intraocular pressure by focusing on certain trabecular meshwork cells. When eye drops are not well tolerated or are ineffective, it is often utilized.

Trabeculoplasty using Argon Laser (ALT):

A further laser technique called ALT improves fluid outflow by opening the eye's drainage angle.

Surgical Procedures:

Trabeculectomy:

A surgical operation called trabeculectomy is used to open up a new conduit for aqueous fluid drainage. This facilitates the decrease of intraocular pressure. The sclera, or white portion of the eye, has a little flap made during this procedure to let fluid escape.

Stents and Shunts:

Shunts: Small channels, or shunts, are made by devices like the Ahmed valve or Baerveldt implant to help drain aqueous humor by rerouting fluid from the eye into a reservoir.

Stents: To enhance the outflow of aqueous humor, tiny implants called intents or Hydrus Microstents are placed into the trabecular meshwork.

When other forms of therapy are unable to sufficiently regulate intraocular pressure, these surgical procedures are often taken into consideration.

Simplified Method Of Solving:

1. Frequent Monitoring: Glaucoma monitoring and early identification depend

heavily on routine eye examinations. Regular examinations assist in early illness detection.

2. Lifestyle Adjustments: Adopting good eating habits and frequent exercise may improve general eye health. According to some research, eating a diet high in antioxidants may provide some protection.

3. Adherence to Medication: Effective treatment depends on patient education and compliance with taking recommended drugs, especially eye drops.

4. Prompt Intervention: Depending on how the condition progresses, laser treatment or surgery may be required. Prompt action may stop more optic nerve injury.

5. Collaborative Care: Ophthalmologists and other medical providers must often work together to effectively treat glaucoma. Follow-ups and regular contact improve the patient's treatment overall.

To sum up, glaucoma treatment is a multimodal strategy that includes everything from drugs and laser therapy to surgery. The severity of the ailment, the patient's reaction to medicine, and other unique characteristics all influence the treatment plan. Effective glaucoma treatment mostly involves patient and healthcare provider collaboration and routine monitoring.

CHAPTER SIX

Adjusting Lifestyle To Manage Glaucoma:

1. Nutrition And Diet:

a. Foods Rich in Antioxidants: - Promote a diet rich in fruits and vegetables, which are high in antioxidants. - Antioxidants that help shield the eyes from oxidative stress include zinc, vitamin C, and vitamin E.

b. Omega-3 Fatty Acids: Consume foods high in omega-3 fatty acids, such as walnuts, flaxseeds, and fish (salmon, mackerel). - The anti-inflammatory qualities of omega-3s may improve eye health.

c. Keep Your Blood Sugar Levels Healthy: - Control your blood sugar levels, particularly if you have diabetes. Uncontrolled diabetes may worsen glaucoma.

d. Drink enough water to prevent dehydration, which might lower intraocular pressure.

2. Physical Activity And Exercise:

a. Regularly do aerobic workouts such as walking, running, or cycling. - Blood circulation is enhanced by exercise, which may lower intraocular pressure.

b. Eye Exercises: To increase the strength and flexibility of your eyes' muscles, do the exercises that eye care specialists prescribe.

c. Yoga: - A few yoga positions and breathing techniques may help lower stress and improve eye health.

3. Handling Stress:

a. Practice mindfulness meditation and other relaxation methods to help you cope with stress. - Prolonged stress may be a factor in high intraocular pressure.

b. Investigate biofeedback methods to take charge of physiological functions and maybe influence intraocular pressure.

c. Interests and Leisure Activities: - Take part in interests and activities that make you happy and calm down to lower your stress levels all around.

4. Suitable Sleep Position:

a. Maintaining a regular sleep pattern is essential to ensuring that you get enough good sleep. - Sleep disorders may worsen the symptoms of glaucoma and have an impact on ocular health.

b. Sleep Position: - If directed by an eye care expert, steer clear of sleeping postures that may raise intraocular pressure.

c. Screen Time Management: - To encourage higher-quality sleep, cut down on screen time before bed.

Making lifestyle changes as part of a comprehensive approach to glaucoma therapy may improve general well-being and perhaps halt the condition's development.

Nonetheless, it is important to seek the opinion of a qualified eye care specialist for customized guidance based on individual requirements and the unique features of glaucoma. For the best possible eye health, medical treatments and routine eye exams should be combined with lifestyle modifications.

CHAPTER SEVEN

Innovations In Technology

Globally, glaucoma—a collection of eye disorders that harm the optic nerve—is one of the main causes of permanent blindness. Appropriate and prompt diagnosis is essential for managing and preventing vision loss.

Modern technology advancements have significantly changed how glaucoma is treated, making it more patient-centered, effective, and accessible. Three main ideas will be covered in this talk: wearable devices for intraocular pressure monitoring, telemedicine and remote monitoring, and artificial intelligence in the diagnosis of glaucoma.

1. Artificial Intelligence In The Diagnosis Of Glaucoma:

The field of healthcare has seen a significant shift in the use of artificial intelligence (AI), and glaucoma diagnosis is no exception. In order to help with the early identification and monitoring of glaucoma, artificial intelligence (AI) algorithms can evaluate complicated information, such as medical imaging and patient records. Here is how AI supports the strategy of streamlined solutions:

Automated Screening: Retinal image analysis using AI-powered systems may identify early indicators of glaucoma, such as alterations in the optic nerve head and faults in the retinal nerve fiber layer, therefore automating the screening procedure. This makes it possible to identify those who are in danger quickly and to intervene when necessary.

Risk Prediction Models: Personalized risk prediction models may be produced by advanced AI algorithms by using different patient variables, including age, genetic propensity, and family history. Healthcare providers may use these models to identify high-risk patients and adjust their treatment strategies appropriately.

Progression Monitoring: AI systems are able to track the advancement of diseases by continually analyzing longitudinal data, such as visual field testing and optic nerve imaging. This guarantees prompt modifications to treatment regimens, halting further loss of eyesight.

2. Remote Monitoring And Telemedicine:

Access to healthcare services has greatly increased with the introduction of telemedicine, especially for those with long-term diseases like glaucoma. Telemedicine-enabled remote monitoring has several advantages for the treatment of glaucoma, including:

Virtual Consultations: Telemedicine eliminates the need for regular in-person visits by enabling patients to consult with eye care specialists from the comfort of their own homes. Those who live in rural or underdeveloped regions will find this to be extremely helpful.

Continuous Monitoring: Real-time data gathering, including medication adherence and intraocular pressure (IOP) readings, is made possible via remote monitoring systems. This ongoing observation improves the accuracy of treatment regimens and makes early intervention easier in the event that deviations occur.

Patient Engagement: Interactive tools and instructional materials are often included in telemedicine systems, enabling patients to take an active role in their own treatment. Better overall results and increased treatment adherence may result from this involvement.

3. Wearable Technology For Monitoring Intraocular Pressure:

Wearable technology provides a practical and non-invasive means of monitoring intraocular pressure, which is important in the treatment of glaucoma. These tools support a method that is more straightforward and patient-friendly:

Continuous IOP Monitoring: Throughout the day, wearable technology—such as intraocular pressure sensors or smart contact lenses—provides continuous IOP monitoring. This information may be easily included in the patient's electronic health record to provide a thorough picture of their health.

Personalized Treatment Plans: Using real-time intraocular pressure data, medical professionals may create customized treatment regimens that take into account each patient's particular intraocular pressure changes. The treatment of glaucoma is more successful when it is customized.

Patient Empowerment: By providing patients with information on their IOP patterns and how lifestyle choices may affect these readings, wearable technology empowers patients. Proactive self-management and a feeling of control are encouraged by this knowledge.

In summary, wearable technology, telemedicine, and artificial intelligence combined with glaucoma management provide a streamlined approach to treatment that improves early identification, remote monitoring, and individualized care. By enabling patients to take an active role in the treatment of their eye health, these technological advancements not only increase the effectiveness of healthcare delivery but also lead to improved results in the battle against glaucoma.

CHAPTER EIGHT

Patient Information And Awareness

A multimodal strategy centered on patient education and awareness is part of a simple solution approach to glaucoma. This strategy is essential for the prompt identification, efficient treatment, and avoidance of visual loss brought on by glaucoma. Let us explore each of these ideas:

1. The Value Of Education For Patients

Comprehending Glaucoma: It is essential to educate patients on the nature of glaucoma, its causes, associated risk factors, and the significance of early diagnosis. People are now more equipped to actively manage their eye health thanks to this information.

Treatment alternatives: Patients should be made aware of all of the alternatives for their care, including prescription drugs, procedures, and lifestyle modifications. Making an educated selection requires knowledge of the possible drawbacks and advantages of various therapies.

Frequent Monitoring: It is critical to emphasize the need for routine eye exams and intraocular pressure monitoring. Patients should be informed that frequent eye examinations are essential for early identification of glaucoma since the condition is often asymptomatic in its early stages.

Medication Compliance: Inform patients of the significance of following their doctors' recommended dosage instructions. The advancement of the illness may be markedly slowed down with regular pharmaceutical usage.

2. Increasing Public Knowledge

Media Campaigns: To spread knowledge about glaucoma, run media campaigns on a variety of venues, including print, radio, social media, and television. To reach a large audience, choose language that is easy to understand.

Community Workshops: Hold seminars in your neighborhood to educate people about glaucoma risk factors, eye health, and the value of routine eye exams. Involve medical specialists in order to provide precise information.

Partnership with Colleges and Schools: Work together with educational establishments to include eye health instruction in the curriculum. Younger populations may become more aware of this and be inspired to start practicing good eye care habits at a young age.

3. Resources And Support Groups

Patient Support Groups: Form and advertise support groups for people with glaucoma diagnoses. Patients may exchange experiences, coping mechanisms, and emotional support in these groups.

Internet Resources: Create and manage glaucoma patient websites with trustworthy information, discussion boards, and resources. This offers a concentrated information source and fosters a feeling of community.

Cooperation with Healthcare professionals: To provide a thorough support system, and encourage cooperation between glaucoma sufferers and healthcare professionals. This might include counseling services, instructional materials, and frequent follow-ups.

To sum up, a simple solution approach to glaucoma includes both active patient education and awareness campaigns in addition to medical treatment. By educating people about glaucoma, raising public awareness, and creating support systems, we may strive toward early identification, better treatment, and an enhanced quality of life for those who are impacted by this disorder that threatens eyesight.

CHAPTER NINE

A Comprehensive Method For Treating Glaucoma

Increased intraocular pressure (IOP) is a common feature of glaucoma, a complicated eye disorder that may cause optic nerve damage and, in the absence of treatment, vision loss. In addition to focusing on the physical symptoms, a holistic approach to glaucoma care blends conventional and alternative treatments, highlights the mind-body link, and customizes treatment regimens to meet the requirements of each patient.

Combining Conventional And Complementary Therapies:

Medication and Surgery: Conventional therapies often include the use of drugs to lower intraocular pressure (eye drops or oral pills) or surgical procedures to enhance fluid outflow. Although these techniques work well, a holistic viewpoint acknowledges that complementary treatments may also be used.

Nutritional Supplements: Research indicates that some supplements, such as omega-3 fatty acids and antioxidants, may help prevent glaucoma. By including them in the therapy regimen, general eye health may be supported.

Herbal treatments and acupuncture: These complementary and alternative therapies have been investigated for their ability to reduce symptoms and enhance ocular circulation. These techniques may be helpful to certain patients, even if scientific data is still developing.

The Mind-Body Link In The Treatment Of Glaucoma:

Stress management: Prolonged stress may be a factor in high intraocular pressure. Deep breathing exercises, mindfulness training, and meditation are among the techniques that might help control stress levels and perhaps improve general eye health.

Biofeedback: People may be trained to regulate physiological processes like heart rate and muscular tension by using biofeedback methods. This may be especially important for controlling glaucoma-related stressors.

Yoga and Tai Chi are examples of mind-body exercises that may improve flexibility, balance, and lower stress levels. Including them in a comprehensive glaucoma treatment plan might improve general health.

Tailored Care Programs:

Customized Evaluation: Since every patient's health is different, a holistic approach includes a detailed evaluation of the patient's lifestyle, stress levels, and general health in addition to their ocular health.

Personalized Lifestyle Recommendations: In order to promote general health and perhaps affect the course of glaucoma, personalized treatment programs may include suggestions for lifestyle alterations including food adjustments, exercise regimens, and sleep hygiene.

Patient education and empowerment: Treatment adherence may be improved by providing patients with information about their disease and allowing them to participate in decision-making. This cooperative method encourages a feeling of responsibility for overseeing their eye health.

In conclusion, by combining conventional and alternative therapies, acknowledging the mind-body link, and customizing treatment regimens to meet each patient's requirements, a holistic approach to glaucoma care surpasses standard treatments. By addressing the underlying causes of glaucoma as well as its symptoms, this all-encompassing approach seeks to improve the general health and well-being of the eyes. In order to create a customized plan that suits their individual needs and preferences, patients must collaborate closely with their healthcare professionals.

Conclusion

To sum up, treating and maintaining glaucoma requires a comprehensive and multimodal approach. In addition to being irreversible, this sight-threatening illness warrants attention since early management has a major impact on results. It is clear from a summary of the main ideas that a simple solution method combines awareness, prompt identification, and an all-encompassing care plan.

Summarizing The Main Ideas:

Comprehending Glaucoma:

A degenerative eye disease called glaucoma is characterized by damage to the optic nerve and is often linked to high intraocular pressure.

Angle-closure glaucoma (acute and abrupt) and open-angle glaucoma (chronic and progressive) are the two basic kinds.

The Value of Prompt Intervention

Because symptoms cannot appear until after severe harm has occurred, early diagnosis is essential.

Early diagnosis depends on routine eye examinations, particularly for those who are more vulnerable (e.g., elderly population, family history).

Early intervention may stop or decrease the progression of vision loss, highlighting the need to raise awareness and do tests on a regular basis.

Options for Treatment:

Surgery, laser therapy, and prescription eye drops are available as treatments.

The kind and severity of glaucoma determine the best course of therapy.

In circumstances when intraocular pressure is advanced, surgical procedures may be considered in addition to medication.

Changes in Lifestyle:

A nutritious diet, frequent exercise, and abstinence from smoking are just a few examples of lifestyle modifications that might improve general eye health.

Systemic diseases such as diabetes and hypertension must be managed since they might affect the course of glaucoma.

Patient Instruction:

Enhancing adherence to treatment programs and lifestyle adjustments requires patient education.

People may take charge of their eye health when they are aware of the chronic nature of glaucoma and the value of regular follow-up visits.

Stressing The Value Of Prompt Intervention:

The cornerstone of managing glaucoma is early intervention. The likelihood of maintaining eyesight is greatly increased by identifying and treating the illness early on. We can all work together to lessen the effects of glaucoma on people and communities by increasing knowledge about the risk factors, advocating for routine eye exams, and fostering proactive behavior when it comes to seeking medical attention.

Promoting A Holistic Approach To The Treatment Of Glaucoma:

Beyond only treating the symptoms, a complete approach to glaucoma treatment addresses the underlying causes, controls risk factors, and offers continuous support. In addition to intraocular pressure, lifestyle variables, concurrent disorders, and specific patient features should be taken into account by healthcare providers. To guarantee a comprehensive and patient-centered approach, cooperation between ophthalmologists, optometrists, primary care doctors, and other healthcare professionals is crucial.

In summary, a thorough care plan, prompt action, and early identification are all part of a simple solution approach to glaucoma. Glaucoma may be lessened and the priceless gift of sight preserved if awareness, education, and a multidisciplinary approach to treatment are given top priority.

THE END

www.ingramcontent.com/pod-product-compliance
Lightning Source LLC
Chambersburg PA
CBHW050748260726
48661CB00001B/482